ECHINACEA

MARIAN KIM

1

PROPERTIES

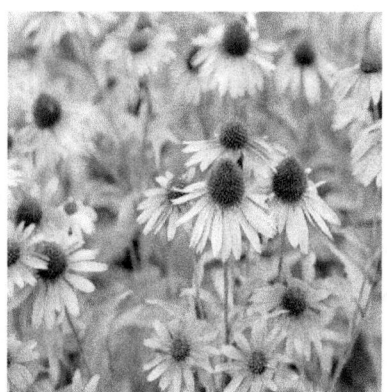

Scientific name: Echinacea purpurea

Other names: American cone flower, black Sampson, black susans, hedgehog, Indian head, Kansas snakeroot

Properties

Immunostimulant (boosts immune system) properties

Anti-inflammatory properties

Antiseptic (antibacterial, antiviral) properties

Depurative (removes waste products from body) properties

Skin regeneration properties

* * * * *

2

USES

Immune system stimulant

Echinacea is used to stimulate the immune system.

Prevent colds

Germany's Commission E (regulatory advisory body) endorses the use of Echinacea purpurea for the treatment of the common cold.

A study done by the University of Connecticut in 2007 revealed that taking 3 grams of dried Echinacea root can reduce the chances of catching a cold by 58%. The duration of the cold was also reduced by 1.4 days. The severity of the cold symptoms was also reduced in persons taking the dried root.

An Echinacea tea to fight colds can be made by steeping the leaves or flowers in boiling water for 20 minutes. This tea should generally be taken at the first sign of a cold. Echinacea tincture is also used for colds. Some herbalists recommend that adults should take 1 dropperful of tincture in water 4 times a day for not more than 10 days. Children should take half the adult's dose.

Fevers

Germany's Commission E (regulatory advisory body) endorses the use of Echinacea purpurea for the treatment of fevers. It is also used to treat other febrile conditions like malaria, diphtheria and typhoid.

Urinary Tract Infections (UTI) Treatment

Germany's Commission E (regulatory advisory body) endorses the use of Echinacea purpurea for the treatment of urinary tract infections.

Burns management

Germany's Commission E (regulatory advisory body) endorses the use of Echinacea purpurea for the treatment of burns. Echinacea salves can be used for this purpose.

Wound and injuries treatment

Echinacea is used to help wounds and minor injuries heal. Echinacea salves can be used for this purpose.

Inset bite and sting treatment

Echinacea is used to help bites and stings from insects like bees heal. Echinacea salves can be used for this purpose.

Snake bite management

Echinacea was originally called snake root because of its restorative effects on persons who had been bitten by rattlesnakes.

Skin infections treatment

Echinacea is used for skin infections like boils. It is also used for inflammatory skin conditions because of its anti-inflammatory properties.

Eczema and psoriasis treatment

Echinacea is used for inflammatory skin conditions like eczema and psoriasis because of its anti-inflammatory properties.

Vaginal yeast infections treatment

Echinacea is used to treat vaginal yeast infections.

Syphilis and genital herpes treatment

Echinacea is used to treat syphilis. It is also used for genital herpes caused by herpes simplex.

Cancer treatment aide

Echinacea is used by patients receiving cancer treatments to reduce the side effects of chemotherapy.

Constipation treatment

Echinacea is as mild laxative since it is a gentle bowel stimulator. It is also used for hemorrhoids and acid indigestion.

Headache treatment

Echinacea is used to relieve the pain of headaches from migraines.

UV radiation skin damage prevention and treatment

Echinacea is used to prevent sunburn and in persons with ultraviolet rays (UV) photo damage it is used to treat it.

Gum disease treatment

Echinacea is used to treat gum disease.

Tonsillitis treatment

Echinacea is used to treat tonsillitis.

Septicemia treatment

Echinacea is used to treat septicemia (bloodstream infections).

Rheumatism treatment

Echinacea is used to treat rheumatism.

Dizziness treatment

Echinacea is used to treat dizziness.

Attention Deficit Hyperactivity Disorder (ADHD) treatment

Echinacea is used to treat ADHD.

Chronic fatigue syndrome treatment

Echinacea is used to treat chronic fatigue syndrome.

*, *, *, *, *

3

SAFETY PRECAUTIONS

1. Echinacea should not be used for long, uninterrupted durations due to its immune stimulating properties. It is generally used for 10 days, discontinued for 1 week and its use continued for 10 more days.

2. Some persons, especially those who are allergic to ragweed and those with hay fever can develop a reaction to Echinacea and develop itchy eyes and throat, hives, nausea and abdominal pain.

3. Persons with autoimmune diseases like systemic lupus erythematosus (lupus, SLE), multiple sclerosis and rheumatoid arthritis should use echinacea with caution and only for the shortest possible duration.

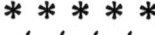

4

DRUG INTERACTIONS

1. Persons taking medications metabolized (broken down) by the liver should not use/avoid Echinacea since it can increase their side effects. Medications metabolized by the liver that might be affected by Echinacea include clarithromycin (Biaxin), cyclosporine (Neoral, Sandimmune), diltiazem (Cardizem), estrogens, haloperidol (Haldol), indinavir (Crixivan), lovastatin (Mevacor), propranolol (Inderal), triazolam (Halcion) and theophylline.

2. Persons taking medications to suppress the immune system (immunosuppresants) should not use Echinacea since it boosts the immune and it will decrease their effectiveness. Examples of immunosuppressants include azathioprine (Imuran), cyclosporine (Neoral, Sandimmune), mycophenolate mofetil (CellCept), tacrolimus (Prograf) and prednisone (Deltasone).

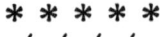

* * * * *

6

HERBAL RECIPES

Echinacea Infusion

Equipment
Glass jar with tight fitting lid

***

Ingredients
1 teaspoon dried Echinacea leaves or flowers or 3 teaspoons fresh Echinacea leaves or flowers

1 cup boiling water

***

Instructions

1. Place the Echinacea in the glass jar and add the boiling water to fill the jar.

2. Close the lid and let the mixture steep for 4 hours to 14 hours (overnight).

3. Strain the Echinacea and the infusion is ready for consumption.

4. Store the infusion in the refrigerator to lengthen its life.

***

Tips

Add 1 teaspoon lemon grass and 1 teaspoon spearmint leaves to make a healing tea for colds.

*****

Echinacea Decoction

Equipment

Non-reactive heavy saucepan

***

Ingredients

1 oz (30 grams) dried Echinacea root

1 pint (500 ml) water

***

Instructions

1. Place the Echinacea and water in the saucepan, cover them and slowly bring the mixture to a simmering boil for 20 minutes.

2. Remove the mixture from the heat source and let the mixture cool to drinking temperature. Strain it, measure and pour the liquid into a clean pan.

3. Heat the liquid until it begins to steam. Reduce the heat and let the liquid continue to steam until it is reduced to half its original volume. This may take 45 minutes to 1 hour.

4. Pour the decoction into a clean bottle.

5. Store the decoction in the refrigerator to lengthen its life.

***

Tips

This decoction can be drunk as a healing tea for colds.

*****

Echinacea Syrup

Equipment

Saucepan

Jar with airtight lid

*

Ingredients

1 quart (1000 ml) filtered water

1 cup dried Echinacea or 3 cups fresh Echinacea

1 cup honey

*

Instructions

1. Place the water and Echinacea in a saucepan and bring to a boil.

2. Reduce the heat and let it simmer while it is partially covered until the volume is reduced to half the original volume.

3. Strain the mixture through a sieve or cheesecloth to remove the Echinacea.

4. Measure 1 pint (500 mls) of the liquid and add the honey.

5. Cook for a few minutes as you stir it so that it thickens.

6. Store the syrup in an airtight container in the fridge for up to 2 months.

**

Echinacea Tincture

Equipment

Glass jar with tight fitting lid

Dark tincture bottles

Cheesecloth

Labels

***

Ingredients

7 oz (200 gm) of dried Echinacea or 14 oz (400 gm) of fresh Echinacea

30 oz (1 liter) of 80-100 proof vodka

***

Instructions

1. Fill 1/3 of the glass jar with the chopped Echinacea.

2. Add the vodka to completely fill the jar to the top.

3. Seal the jar and label it with the date of preparation and name of Echinacea used.

4. Store the glass jar in a dark place for 6 weeks ensuring that you shake them weekly.

5. After 6 weeks strain out the Echinacea with a cheesecloth and pour the tincture into dark tincture bottles.

6. Label the tincture bottles with the date and name of Echinacea used.

7. Store your herbal tinctures away from light and heat.

*****

Echinacea Poultice

Equipment

Cheesecloth or old cotton sheet strips

***

Ingredients

1 tablespoon powdered dry Echinacea

Boiling water

***

Instructions

1. Add enough boiling water to the Echinacea to wet it and make a thick paste.

2. Spoon the Echinacea paste onto the cheesecloth (or bed sheet strips) to make the poultice.

3. To use, apply the poultice to the affected area and cover with another piece of hot, wet cloth. Replace the hot, wet cloth when it cools with another hot one to keep the poultice hot.

*****

Echinacea Infused Oil

Equipment

Double boiler

Large glass bowl

Sieve and cheesecloth

Sterilized dark jars

***

Ingredients

16 fl oz. (500 ml) pure vegetable oils like organic olive oil, sweet almond oil or sunflower oil

8 oz. (250 grams) dry Echinacea powder or 16 oz. (500 grams) slightly bruised, fresh Echinacea

***

Instructions

1. Place the Echinacea and oil in the glass bowl ensuring that the oil covers the Echinacea. Simmer them in a double boiler for one hour at a temperature of around 120 degrees Fahrenheit (49 degrees Celsius). Do not let the mixture boil. You can repeat this step several times after letting the oils cool to create more concentrated herb infused oils.

2. Strain the mixture through the sieve and cheesecloth into a clean, dark jar ensuring you squeeze out as much oil as you can from the cheesecloth.

3. Label your jars with the manufacturing date, expiry date, Echinacea and oils used.

4. Store your Echinacea infused oils in a cool dark place or in the refrigerator and use them within 3 months.

*****

Echinacea Salve

Equipment

Double boiler

Large glass bowl

Sterilized dark jars or tins

***

Ingredients

8 oz. (250 ml or 1 cup) Echinacea infused vegetable oil (see previous recipe)

1 oz. (30 grams) beeswax

10 drops essential oils like lavender essential oil (optional natural fragrance)

***

Instructions

1. Place the beeswax and Echinacea infused oil in the glass bowl and melt them in a double boiler.

2. Once melted remove from the heat source, allow to cool and add the essential oils (if using).

3. Pour the melted oils into the storage jars or tins and allow to cool completely.

4. Store the salves in a cool dark place.

###

ABOUT THE AUTHOR

Marian Kim is an experienced alternative medicine practitioner.

OTHER BOOKS BY THE AUTHOR

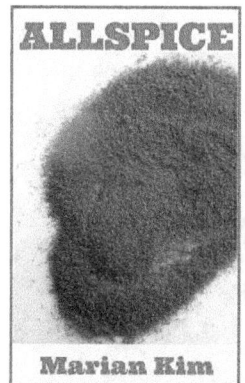

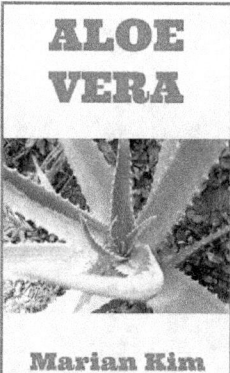

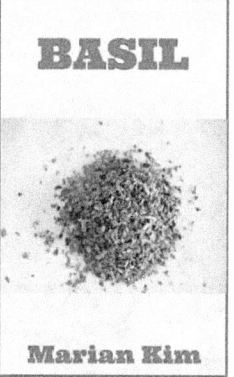

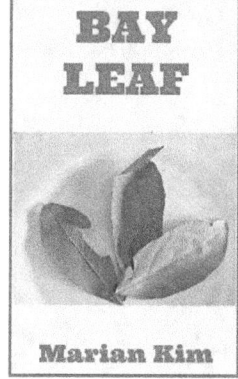

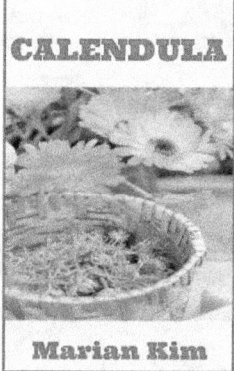

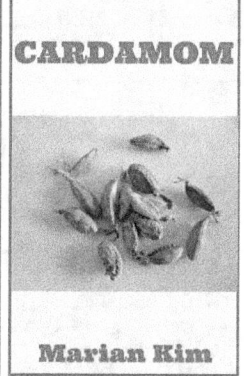

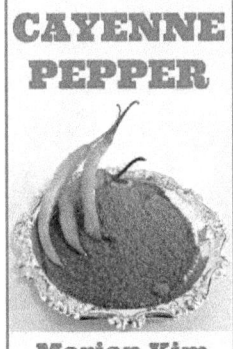

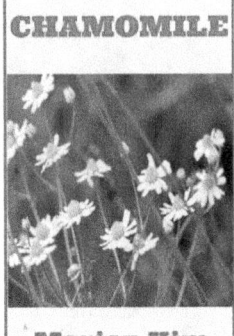

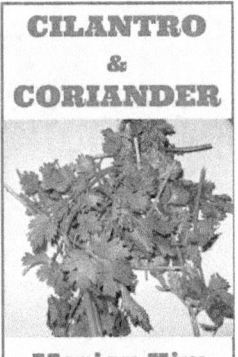

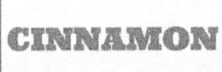

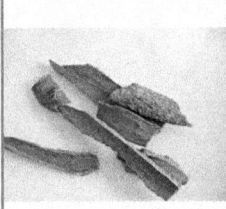

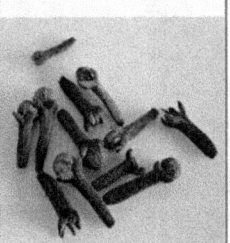

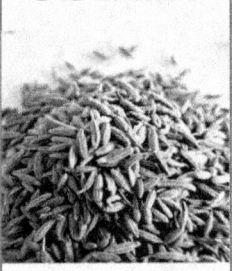

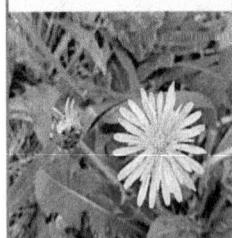

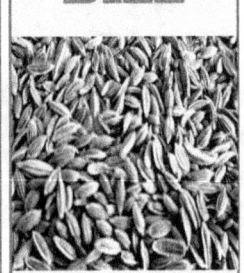

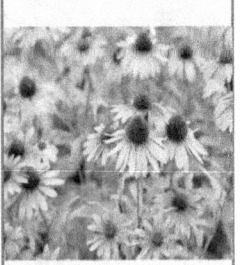

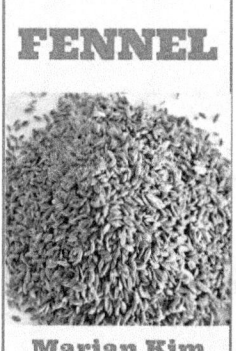

FENNEL

Marian Kim

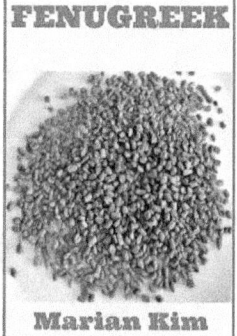

FENUGREEK

Marian Kim

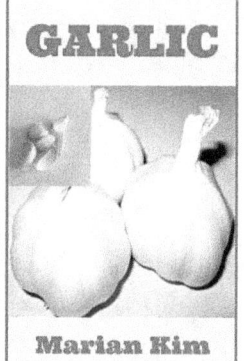

GARLIC

Marian Kim

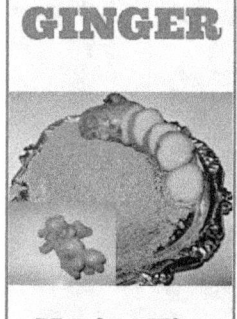

GINGER

Marian Kim

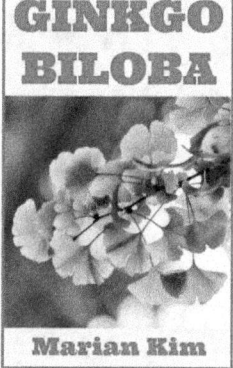

GINKGO BILOBA

Marian Kim

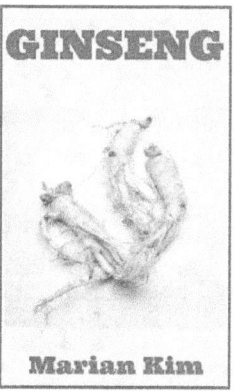

GINSENG

Marian Kim

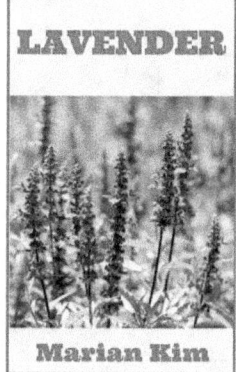

LAVENDER

Marian Kim

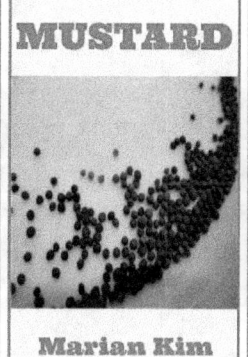

MUSTARD

Marian Kim

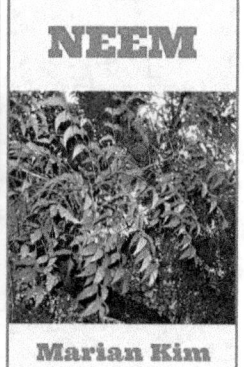

NEEM

Marian Kim

NUTMEG & MACE

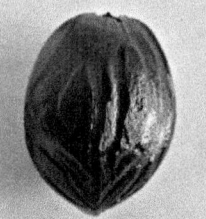

Marian Kim

OREGANO

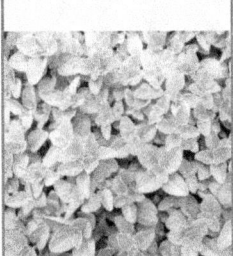

Marian Kim

PAPRIKA

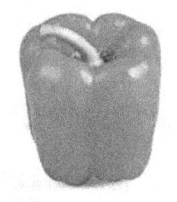

Marian Kim

PARSLEY

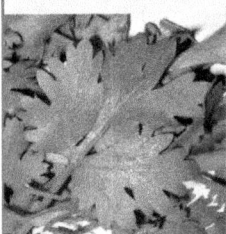

Marian Kim

BLACK & WHITE PEPPER

Marian Kim

PEPPERMINT

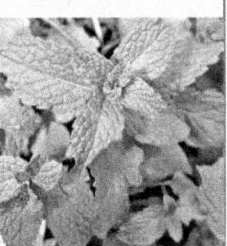

Marian Kim

ROSE HIPS

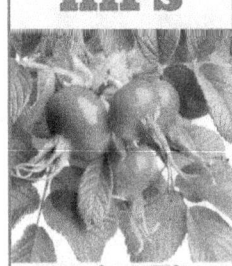

Marian Kim

ROSE PETALS

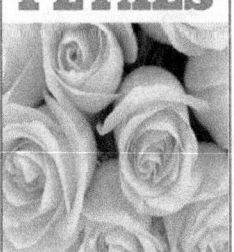

Marian Kim

ROSEMARY

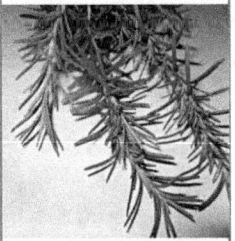

Marian Kim

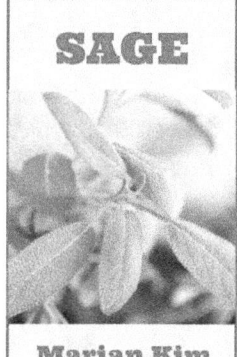

SAGE

Marian Kim

ST. JOHN'S WORT

Marian Kim

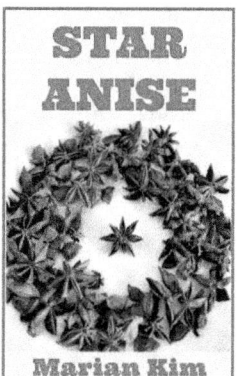

STAR ANISE

Marian Kim

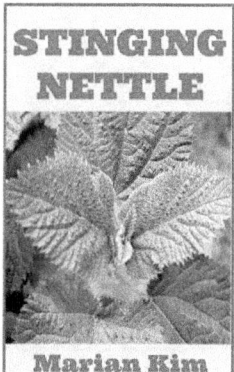

STINGING NETTLE

Marian Kim

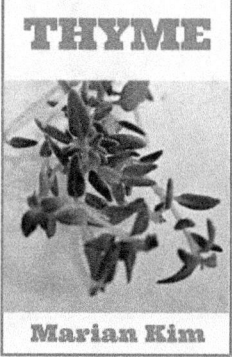

THYME

Marian Kim

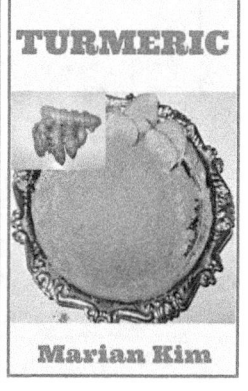

TURMERIC

Marian Kim

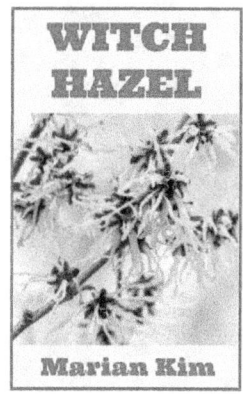

WITCH HAZEL

Marian Kim

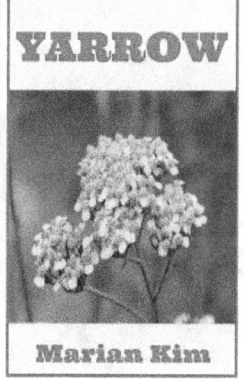

YARROW

Marian Kim

*****